Dash Diet Meal Plan

Easy Delicious Low-Calorie Recipes With Complete 21-Day Eating Plan To Drop Extra Weight, Boost Metabolism, Increase Energy Levels And Get Healthy Fast

Mary Stone

Table of Contents

Introduction

The DASH Diet is a diet used to lower blood pressure. It is also known as DASH (Dietary Approaches to Stop Hypertension). This diet is primarily used to treat people with high blood pressure, but has also been shown to be effective for certain complications of diabetes, and may also reduce the risk of heart disease.

The DASH diet encourages the consumption of nutrient-rich foods that are also lower in energy. When following this diet, 2,000 calories a day assume the use of a food totaling system.

This diet, due to its low content of saturated fat and its high content of fruit and vegetables, promotes the reduction of heart disease. It can be especially helpful for controlling the amount of sodium consumed per day, and reducing the risk of strokes and high blood pressure.

The guidelines of DASH are mainly aimed at reducing the amount of salt consumed. In fact, salt is eliminated as completely as possible or at least reduced. There is a limited number of low-fat products, white bread and rice that can be consumed.

It is not only the salt, but also the fat consumption that is limited on this diet. It is primarily aimed at reducing blood pressure and cholesterol. It was introduced in 1993 by the National Heart, Lung, and Blood Institute.

The diet is not designed to be followed as long as the others. It is a diet to think of as a solution to a possible dietary problem in the long term and therefore for a limited period of time. There is no fixed period for which this diet is to be followed.

In general, the DASH diet provides for a lower amount of salt, saturated fat, and cholesterol in the body. This is achieved by a lowering of blood pressure and by a regulation of the other substances. It is also necessary to have the approval of the physician.

This diet is very low in sodium and permits a moderate amount of potassium. The food is primarily based on vegetable or low-density fruits and grains, cereals, poultry and fish. There is a reduction in sodium and carbohydrates which are rich in vitamins and minerals, sweets and alcohol, white bread and rice, and dairy products.

Dash Diet has gained popularity in the past few years as it is extremely helpful in strengthening metabolism and controlling hypertension. Contrary to the popular belief that while following the dash diet, one gets to only eat vegetarian foods while you get a balanced diet that includes fresh fruits, vegetables, nuts, low-fat dairy products and whole grains. You do not have to completely cut down on meat; instead you just have to reduce sodium and fat content from your everyday diet.

The diet also has many health benefits as it helps in reducing hypertension and obesity lowering osteoporosis and preventing cancer. This well-balanced diet strengthens metabolism which further helps in decomposing the fat deposits stored in the body. This, in turn, enhances the general health of a person.

This diet is easy to follow as you get to everything but in a healthier fashion and limited quantity.

CHAPTER 1:

What Is the DASH Diet?

Endorsed by the United States National Heart, Lung, and Blood Institute, the DASH (Dietary Approaches to Stop Hypertension) diet studies the nutrient composition of food items to prepare unique dietary strategies that help to reduce high blood pressure. The diet is a result of the engineering done by bio-scientists and lawmakers to find the components that must be eliminated from one's diet to control the rise of blood pressure.

The DASH diet came about because the number of people complaining of high blood pressure almost doubled in the last two decades. This led medical experts, along with the United States Department of Health and Human Services, to find ways to deal with hypertension and eliminate the various risks that are associated with high blood pressure. After a careful study, the researchers found that people who prefer to consume more vegetables or who followed a plant-based diet showed fewer signs and cases of rising blood pressure. This, therefore, became the foundation of the DASH diet.

In the DASH diet, the person focuses on consuming foods that are non-processed and more organic. Whole grains, fruits, vegetables, and lean meats form the essential components of this diet technique. In extreme cases, the person showing major signs of heart-related ailments due to high blood pressure is also advised to go vegan for some time to lower issues related to hypertension.

The diet also follows a strict method of using salt. Because too much salt and oil significantly raise the blood pressure in the human body, the dietary guidelines of the DASH diet significantly reduce the intake of salt. The recipes in the DASH diet are a wholesome mix of green vegetables, natural fruits, low-fat dairy foods, and lean protein such as chicken, fish, and a lot of beans. Besides limiting the intake of salt, the rule of thumb is to minimize food items rich in red meat, processed sugars, and composite fat. As per the standard practice, anyone following the DASH diet is advised not to consume more than one teaspoon (2,300 mg) of sodium in a day.

The diet is safe to follow and is also accredited by the United States Department of Agriculture (USDA). The US Dietary Guidelines also included the DASH diet as one of three healthy diets recommended in 2015-2020.

Benefits of the DASH diet

The benefits of the DASH diet go beyond reducing hypertension and heart ailments.

Controlling blood pressure: The force exerted on our blood vessels and organs when the blood passes through them is a measure of blood pressure in the human body. When blood pressure increases beyond a certain level, it can lead to various bodily malfunctions, including heart failure.

Blood pressure is counted in two numbers: systolic pressure (pressure exerted in the blood vessels when the heart beats) and diastolic pressure (pressure exerted in the blood vessels when the heart is at rest). The normal blood systolic pressure in adults is below 120 mmHg, while the diastolic pressure is typically below 80 mmHg. Anyone over these limits is said to be suffering from high blood pressure.

CHAPTER 2:

What to Eat and Avoid on Dash Diet

Grain Products

What to eat	Eat occasionally	What to avoid
Brown rice	Whole-wheat pasta	White rice
Whole-grain breakfast cereals	Whole-wheat noodles	Regular pasta
Bulgur		White bread
Quinoa		
Oatmeal		
Popcorn		
Rice cakes		

Use only whole grains because they are richer in fiber and nutrients. They are low-fat and can easily substitute butter, cheese, and cream.

Vegetables

What to eat	What to avoid
All fresh vegetables and greens	Regular canned vegetables
Low-sodium canned vegetables	

Vegetables are the richest source of fiber, vitamins, potassium, and magnesium. You can use vegetables not only as a side dish but also as a topping, spread, or meat-free main dish substitutes.

Fruits and Berries

Fruits and berries have the same vital benefits as vegetables. They are rich in minerals and vitamins.

One more advantage of fruits and berries is their low-fat content. They can be a good substitution for desserts and snacks. 0

Fruit peels contain the highest amount of fiber and useful nutrients in comparison with fruit flesh.

What to eat	Eat occasionally	What to avoid
All fruits and berries (pineapple, apple, mango, pears, strawberries, raspberries, dates, apricots, etc.)	Grapefruit Orange Lemon	Sugar added canned fruits Coconut

Dairy

Dairy products are the main source of D vitamins and calcium. The only restriction for dash diet followers is saturated and high-fat dairy products.

Note: you can substitute dairy products with nut, almond, cashew, and soy milk.

What to eat	Eat occasionally	What to avoid
Low-fat or fat-free cheese Low-fat or fat-free yogurt Low-fat or fat-free milk/percent milk Low-fat or fat-free skim milk Low-fat or fat-free frozen yogurt	Low-fat cream Low-fat buttermilk	Full-fat cream Full-fat milk Full-fat cheese Full-fat yogurt

Meat and Poultry

Meat is rich in zinc, B vitamins, protein, and iron. There is a wide variety of recipes that will help you to cook meat in different ways. You can broil, grill, bake or roast it but anyways it will be delicious.
Note: avoid to eat skin and fat from poultry and meat.

What to eat	Eat occasionally	What to avoid
Skinless chicken breast	Lean cuts of red meat (pork, beef, veal, lamb)	Fat cuts of meat
Skinless chicken thighs	Eggs	Pork belly
Skinless chicken wings		Bacon
Skinless drumsticks		Fat
Chicken fillet		

Fish and Seafood
The main benefits you will get from the fish which is high in omega-3 fatty acids. All types of seafood and fish are allowed on the dash diet. You will find the best fish choice for the dash diet below.

What to eat	What to avoid
Salmon	High sodium canned fish and seafood
Herring	
Tuna	

Nuts, Seeds, and Legumes
This type of product is rich in fiber, phytochemicals, potassium, magnesium, and proteins. It has the ability to fight cancer and cardiovascular disease.
Nuts, seeds, and legumes are high in calories and should be eaten in moderation. Add them into your salads or main dishes, they will saturate the taste.

What to eat
All types of seeds
All types of nuts
All types of legumes

Fats and Oils
The main function of fats is to help in absorbing vitamins; nevertheless, the high amount of fats can lead to developing heart diseases, obesity, and diabetes.

According to the dash diet, your daily meal plan shouldn't include more than 30% of fats of daily calories.

What to eat	Eat occasionally	What to avoid
Margarine	Low-fat mayonnaise	Butter
Vegetable oils	Light-salad dressings	Lard
		Solid shortening
		Palm oil

Sweets

It is not necessary to cross out all sweets from your daily diet but it is important to follow some restrictions that the dash diet provides: choose sugar-free, low-fat/fat-free sweets or replace them with fruits and berries.

What to eat	Eat occasionally		What to avoid
Fruit/berries	Hard candy		Biscuits
sorbets	Splenda		Crackers
Fruit ice	Aspartame	(NutraSweet,	Cookies
Graham crackers	Equal)		Soda
Honey	Agave syrup		Unrefined
Sugar-free fruit jelly	Maple syrup		sugar
			Table sugar
			Sweet junk
			food

Alcohol and Caffeine

You should limit alcohol to 2 drinks per day for men and up to 1 or fewer drinks for women.

Note: alcohol and caffeine consumption can be forbidden totally if it is required according to a medical examination.

CHAPTER 3:

Tips for DASH Diet Success

Make a list before going to the store. Often, we don't plan before going to the grocery store. This can result in buying more food than you needed and getting distracted by non-healthy foods that aren't right for the DASH diet. Find healthy and delicious DASH diet recipes beforehand and write down all the ingredients you need. You won't be tempted by the other food in the grocery store because your mind will be set on the delicious meals you've already thought of that are in agreement with the DASH diet rules.

Eat before going shopping. Similar to the last tip, never shop hungry. When you're hungry you have a wandering eye that will want to eat more than what's on your list. Also, when you're hungry you may gravitate towards snacks and processed foods for a quick fix to your hunger. Processed foods are a big no for the DASH diet since they're often high in sodium, so avoid the temptations by not shopping when you're hungry.

Keep *DASH-approved* food at home. Diets are all about avoiding temptation. When you keep junk food and sweets around next to your healthy options, you're more likely to pick the former. However, if you have the basic DASH food staples, like grains, vegetables, nuts, and fruit you're more likely to eat these out of convenience, rather than leave to go to the store and indulge in junk food. Out of sight, out of mind.

Cook's wear is important to consider. Certain tools in the kitchen will be more beneficial to the DASH diet than others. Here are three kitchen cook wear items that you should have in your kitchen. The first is a nonstick pan. This eliminated the need to coat the pan with oil or butter. Since oils and fats are low on the list of food groups you should be eating, it's best to cut down on these fats when you can.

Next, a steamer. Steamers are great because all it adds to your DASH-approved vegetable is water. Healthy food is cooked to perfection. Lastly, a spice mill to grind up whole, natural spices so you avoid livening up your meals with salt.

Rinse off canned foods. Canned vegetables are a quick way to buy vegetables, prepare them, and have them last. They're perfectly okay to eat under the DASH diet. However, the juice in the can carries a lot of excess salt. Get rid of most of this excess by simply rinsing your vegetables off with water before you eat them.

Don't be afraid to ask. It can feel difficult to go out to eat and still maintain your diet. If you want to order something off the menu but are afraid that the salt content may be too high, ask the waiter to ask the chef. Many people have dietary restrictions and you're not a burden for asking. This way, you can eat guilt-free and enjoy your meal. Also, check the ingredients. If the menu doesn't list all of the ingredients on the page, ask your waiter. They may have to ask the chef or sometimes a deeper nutritional value of each item is available on the restaurant's website.

Drink only water. This is a hard feat for some and an easy one for others. If you're a big soda or juice fan, this tip is for you. Sugars, even "fake sugars" like Splenda are put into common prepackaged drinks. Even when buying juice, you may think it'll be fine because it's a serving of your fruit intake for the day. This may be true, however there may also be so many added sugars to the drink that the one fruit serving was ultimately canceled out by the influx of sugar in the juice. You can even branch out to sparkling water or tea but steer clear of drinks with hidden sugars.

Ask for the lunch portion. It's important with the DASH diet to keep your calories at the respected amount. Often at restaurants, a large portion is given and when it's on your plate, your mind feels obligated to eat it. Ask for the lunch portion if you're out to dinner and have them put the rest in a to-go box. Not only are you sticking with your diet this way, but you also are saving money with an extra portion for later.

CHAPTER 4:

Breakfast

1.   Shrimp Skillet

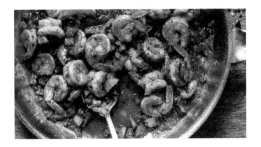

Preparation time: 10 minutes

Cooking time: 25 minutes

Servings: 5

Ingredients:

- 2 bell peppers

- 1 red onion

- 1-pound shrimps, peeled

- ½ teaspoon ground coriander

- ½ teaspoon white pepper

- ½ teaspoon paprika

- 1 tablespoon butter

Directions:

1. Remove the seeds from the bell peppers and cut the vegetable into the wedges.

2. Then place them in the skillet.

3. Add peeled shrimps, white pepper, paprika, and butter.

4. Peel and slice the red onion. Add it in the skillet too.

5. Preheat the oven to 365f.

6. Cover the skillet with foil and secure the edges.

7. Transfer it in the preheated oven and cook for 20 minutes.

8. When the time is over, discard the foil and cook the dish for 5 minutes more -use ventilation mode if you have.

Nutrition: calories 153, fat 4, fiber 1.3, carbs 7.3, protein 21.5

2. Coconut Yogurt with Chia Seeds

Preparation time: 2 hours

Cooking time: 10 minutes

Servings: 4

Ingredients:

- 1 probiotic capsule -yogurt capsule

- 1 cup of coconut milk

- 1 tablespoon coconut meat

- 4 tablespoons chia seeds

Directions:

1. Pour coconut milk in the saucepan and preheat it till 108F.

2. Then add a probiotic capsule and stir well. Close the lid and leave the coconut milk for 40 minutes.

3. Meanwhile, shred coconut meat.

4. When the time is over, transfer the almond milk mixture into the cheesecloth and squeeze it. Leave it like this for 40 minutes more or until the liquid from yogurt is squeezed.

5. After this, transfer the yogurt into the serving glasses.

6. Add chia seeds and coconut meat in every glass and mix up well.

7. Let the cooked yogurt rest for 10 minutes before serving.

Nutrition: calories 177, fat 16.9, fiber 3.9, carbs 6.5, protein 2.6

3.   Chia Pudding

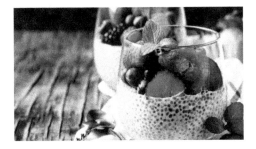

Preparation time: 15 minutes

Cooking time: 3 minutes

Servings: 4

Ingredients:

- 2 cups almond milk

- 8 tablespoons chia seeds

- 1 oz blackberries

- 1 tablespoon Erythritol

Directions:

1. Preheat almond milk for 3 minutes, then remove it from the heat and add chia seeds.

2. Stir gently and add Erythritol. Mix it up.

3. In the bottom of serving glasses put blackberries.

4. Then pour almond milk mixture over berries. Let the pudding rest for at least 10 minutes before serving.

Nutrition: calories 331, fat 31.9, fiber 6.7, carbs 11.8, protein 4.6

4.   Egg Fat Bombs

Preparation time: 10 minutes

Cooking time: 10 minutes

Servings: 4

Ingredients:

- 4 oz bacon, sliced

- 4 eggs, boiled

- 1 tablespoon butter, softened

- ½ teaspoon salt

- ½ teaspoon ground black pepper

- 1 tablespoon mayonnaise

Directions:

1. Line the tray with the baking paper. Place the bacon on the paper.

2. Preheat the oven to 365F and put the tray inside.

3. Cook the bacon for 10 minutes or until it is light brown.

4. Meanwhile, peeled and chop the boiled eggs and transfer them in the mixing bowl.

5. ADD GROUND BLACK PEPPER, MAYONNAISE, AND SALT.

6. When the bacon is cooked, chill it little and finely chop.

7. Add bacon in the egg mixture. Stir it well.

8. Add softened butter and mix up it again.

9. With the help of the scoop make medium size balls. Before serving, place them in the fridge for 10 minutes.

Nutrition: calories 255, fat 20.3, fiber 0.1, carbs 1.2, protein 16.1

5.   Morning "Grits"

Preparation time: 10 minutes

Cooking time: 10 minutes

Servings: 4

Ingredients:

- 1 ½ cup almond milk

- 1 cup heavy cream, whipped

- 4 tablespoon chia seeds

- 3 oz Parmesan, grated

- ½ teaspoon chili flakes

- ½ teaspoon salt

- 1 tablespoon butter

Directions:

1. Pour almond milk in the saucepan and bring it to boil.

2. Meanwhile, grind the chia seeds with the help of the coffee grinder.

3. Remove the almond milk from the heat and add grinded chia seeds.

4. Add whipped cream, chili flakes, and salt. Stir it well and leave for 5 minutes.

5. After this, add butter and grated parmesan. Stir well and preheat it over the low heat until the cheese is melted.

6. Stir it again and transfer in the serving bowls.

Nutrition: calories 439, fat 42.2, fiber 4.4, carbs 9.6, protein 10.7

6.   Scotch Eggs

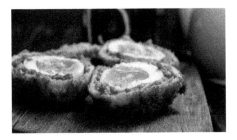

Preparation time: 15 minutes

Cooking time: 15 minutes

Servings: 4

Ingredients:

- 4 eggs, boiled

- 1 ½ cup ground beef

- 1 tablespoon onion, grated

- ½ teaspoon ground black pepper

- ½ teaspoon salt

- ½ teaspoon dried oregano ½ teaspoon dried basil

- 1 tablespoon butter ¾ cup of water

Directions:

1. In the mixing bowl, mix up together ground beef, grated onion, ground black pepper, salt, dried oregano, and basil.

2. Peel the boiled eggs.

3. Make 4 balls from the ground beef mixture.

4. Put peeled eggs inside every ground beef ball and press them gently to get the shape of eggs.

5. Spread the tray with the butter and place ground beef eggs on it.

6. Add water.

7. Preheat oven to 365F and transfer the tray inside.

8. Cook the dish for 15 minutes or until each side of Scotch eggs is light brown.

Nutrition: calories 188, fat 13.4, fiber 0.2, carbs 0.9, protein 15.4

7. Bacon Sandwich

Preparation time: 15 minutes

Cooking time: 20 minutes

Servings: 2

Ingredients:

- 1 oz bacon, sliced -4 slices
- 4 eggs, separated
- 2 teaspoons ricotta cheese
- ¾ teaspoon cream of tartar
- 1 teaspoon flax meal, ground
- 2 lettuce leaves

Directions:

1. Whisk the eggs yolks with 1 teaspoon of ricotta cheese until you get a soft and light fluffy mixture.

2. After this, whip together egg whites with remaining ricotta cheese, salt, and cream of tartar. When the mixture is fluffy, add ground flax meal and stir gently.

3. Preheat the oven to 310F.

4. Gently combine together egg yolk mixture and egg white mixture.

5. Line the tray with baking paper.

6. Make the 4 medium size clouds from the egg mixture using the spoon.

7. Transfer the tray in the oven and cook them for 20 minutes or until they are light brown.

8. Meanwhile, place bacon slices in the skillet and roast them for 1 minute from each side over the medium-high heat.

9. Chill the bacon little.

10. Transfer the cooked and chilled egg clouds on the plate.

11. Place bacon onto 2 clouds and then add lettuce leaves. Cover them with the remaining egg clouds.

12. Secure the sandwiches with toothpicks and transfer in the serving plate.

Nutrition: calories 218, fat 15.5, fiber 0.4, carbs 2.3, protein 17.2

8.   Noatmeal

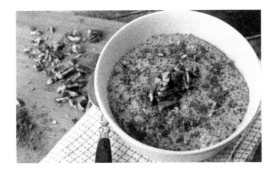

Preparation time: 10 minutes

Cooking time: 10 minutes

Servings: 3

Ingredients:

- 1 cup organic almond milk

- 2 tablespoons hemp seeds

- 1 tablespoon chia seeds, dried

- 1 tablespoon Erythritol

- 1 tablespoon almond flakes

- 2 tablespoons coconut flour

- 1 tablespoon flax meal

- 1 tablespoon walnuts, chopped

- ½ teaspoon vanilla extract

- ¼ teaspoon ground cinnamon

Directions:

1. Put all the ingredients except vanilla extract in the saucepan and stir gently.

2. Cook the mixture on the low heat for 10 minutes. Stir it constantly.

3. When the mixture starts to be thick, add vanilla extract. Mix it up.

4. Remove the noatmeal from the heat and let it rest little.

Nutrition: calories 350, fat 30.4, fiber 8.4, carbs 16.9, protein 9.1

9.   Breakfast Bake with Meat

Preparation time: 10 minutes

Cooking time: 30 minutes

Servings: 4

Ingredients:

- 1 cup ground beef

- 1 cup cauliflower, shredded

- ½ cup coconut cream

- 1 onion, diced

- 1 teaspoon butter

- ½ teaspoon salt

- ½ teaspoon paprika

- ½ teaspoon garam masala

- 1 tablespoon fresh cilantro, chopped

- 1 oz celery root, grated

- 1 oz Cheddar cheese, grated

Directions:

1. Mix up together garam masala mixture, celery root, paprika, salt, and ground beef.

2. Mix up together shredded cauliflower and salt.

3. Spread the casserole tray with butter.

4. Make the layer of the ground beef mixture inside the casserole tray.

5. Then place the layer of the cauliflower mixture and diced onion.

6. Sprinkle it with grated cheese and fresh cilantro, Add coconut cream.

7. Cover the surface of the casserole with the foil and secure the lids.

8. Preheat the oven to 365F.

9. Place the casserole tray in the oven and cook it for 30 minutes.

10. When the time is over, transfer the casserole from the oven, remove the foil and let it chill for 15 minutes.

11. Cut it into the serving and transfer in the serving bowls.

Nutrition: calories 192, fat 14.7, fiber 2.1, carbs 6.5, protein 10

10.   Breakfast Bagel

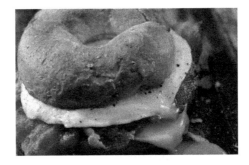

Preparation time: 15 minutes

Cooking time: 30 minutes

Servings: 3

Ingredients:

- ½ cup almond flour

- 1 ½ teaspoon xanthan gum

- 1 egg, beaten

- 3 oz Parmesan, grated

- ½ teaspoon cumin seeds

- 1 teaspoon cream cheese

- 1 teaspoon butter, melted

Directions:

1. In the mixing bowl, mix up together almond flour, xanthan gum, and egg.

2. Stir it until homogenous.

3. Put the cheese in the separate bowl, add cream cheese.

4. Microwave the mixture until it is melted. Stir it well.

5. Combine together cheese mixture and almond flour mixture and knead the dough.

6. Roll the dough into the log.

7. Cut the log into 3 pieces and make bagels.

8. Line the tray with baking paper and place bagels on it.

9. Brush the meal with melted butter and sprinkle with cumin seeds.

10. Preheat the oven to 365F.

11. Put the tray with bagels in the oven and cook 30 minutes.

12. Check if the bagels are cooked with the help of the toothpicks.

13. Cut the bagels and spread them with your favorite spread.

Nutrition: calories 262, fat 18.6, fiber 8.7, carbs 12, protein 15.1

CHAPTER 5:

Lunch

11.   Juicy and Peppery Tenderloin

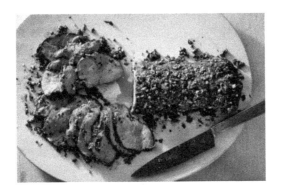

Preparation time: 10 minutes

Cooking time: 20 minutes

Servings: 4

Ingredients:

- 2 teaspoons sage, chopped

- Sunflower seeds and pepper

- 2 1/2 pounds beef tenderloin

- 2 teaspoons thyme, chopped

- 2 garlic cloves, sliced

- 2 teaspoons rosemary, chopped

- 4 teaspoons olive oil

Directions:

1. Preheat your oven to 425 degrees F.

2. Take a small knife and cut incisions in the tenderloin; insert one slice of garlic into the incision.

3. Rub meat with oil.

4. Take a bowl and add sunflower seeds, sage, thyme, rosemary, pepper and mix well.

5. Rub the spice mix over tenderloin.

6. Put rubbed tenderloin into the roasting pan and bake for 10 minutes.

7. Lower temperature to 350 degrees F and cook for 20 minutes more until an internal thermometer reads 145 degrees F.

8. Transfer tenderloin to a cutting board and let sit for 15 minutes; slice into 20 pieces and enjoy!

Nutrition:

Calorie: 183, Fat: 9g, Carbohydrates: 1g, Protein: 24g

12.　Healthy Avocado Beef Patties

Preparation time: 15 minutes

Cooking time: 10 minutes

Servings: 2

Ingredients:

- 1 pound 85% lean ground beef

- 1 small avocado, pitted and peeled

- Fresh ground black pepper as needed

Directions:

1. Pre-heat and prepare your broiler to high.

2. Divide beef into two equal-sized patties.

3. Season the patties with pepper accordingly.

4. Broil the patties for 5 minutes per side.

5. Transfer the patties to a platter.

6. Slice avocado into strips and place them on top of the patties.

7. Serve and enjoy!

Nutrition:

Calories: 568, Fat: 43g, Net Carbohydrates: 9g, Protein: 38g

13. Ravaging Beef Pot Roast

Preparation time: 10 minutes

Cooking time: 75 minutes

Servings: 4

Ingredients:

- 3 ½ pounds beef roast

- 4 ounces mushrooms, sliced

- 12 ounces beef stock

- 1-ounce onion soup mix

- ½ cup Italian dressing, low sodium, and low fat

Directions:

1. Take a bowl and add the stock, onion soup mix and Italian dressing.

2. Stir.

3. Put beef roast in pan.

4. Add mushrooms, stock mix to the pan and cover with foil.

5. Preheat your oven to 300 degrees F.

6. Bake for 1 hour and 15 minutes.

7. Let the roast cool.

8. Slice and serve.

9. Enjoy with the gravy on top!

Nutrition:

Calories: 700, Fat: 56g, Carbohydrates: 10g, Protein: 70g

14. Lovely Faux Mac and Cheese

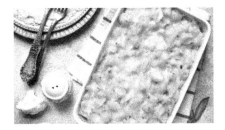

Preparation time: 15 minutes

Cooking time: 45 minutes

Servings: 4

Ingredients:

- 5 cups cauliflower florets

- Sunflower seeds and pepper to taste

- 1 cup coconut almond milk

- ½ cup vegetable broth

- 2 tablespoons coconut flour, sifted

- 1 organic egg, beaten

- 1 cup cashew cheese

Directions:

1. Preheat your oven to 350 degrees F.

2. Season florets with sunflower seeds and steam until firm.

3. Place florets in a greased ovenproof dish.

4. Heat coconut almond milk over medium heat in a skillet, make sure to season the oil with sunflower seeds and pepper.

5. Stir in broth and add coconut flour to the mix, stir.

6. Cook until the sauce begins to bubble.

7. Remove heat and add beaten egg.

8. Pour the thick sauce over the cauliflower and mix in cheese.

9. Bake for 30-45 minutes.

10. Serve and enjoy!

Nutrition:

Calories: 229; Fat: 14g; Carbohydrates: 9g; Protein: 15g

15.   Epic Mango Chicken

Preparation time: 25 minutes

Cooking time: 10 minutes

Servings: 4

Ingredients:

- 2 medium mangoes, peeled and sliced

- 10-ounce coconut almond milk

- 4 teaspoons vegetable oil

- 4 teaspoons spicy curry paste

- 14-ounce chicken breast halves, skinless and boneless, cut in cubes

- 4 medium shallots

- 1 large English cucumber, sliced and seeded

Directions:

1. Slice half of the mangoes and add the halves to a bowl.

2. Add mangoes and coconut almond milk to a blender and blend until you have a smooth puree.

3. Keep the mixture on the side.

4. Take a large-sized pot and place it over medium heat, add oil and allow the oil to heat up.

5. Add curry paste and cook for 1 minute until you have a nice fragrance, add shallots and chicken to the pot and cook for 5 minutes.

6. Pour mango puree in to the mix and allow it to heat up.

7. Serve the cooked chicken with mango puree and cucumbers.

8. Enjoy!

Nutrition:

Calories: 398; Fat: 20g; Carbohydrates: 32g; Protein: 26g

16.   Chicken and Cabbage Platter

Preparation time: 9 minutes

Cooking time: 14 minutes

Servings: 2

Ingredients:

- ½ cup sliced onion

- 1 tablespoon sesame garlic-flavored oil

- 2 cups shredded Bok-Choy

- 1/2 cups fresh bean sprouts

- 1 1/2 stalks celery, chopped

- 1 ½ teaspoons minced garlic

- 1/2 teaspoon stevia

- 1/2 cup chicken broth

- 1 tablespoon coconut aminos

- 1/2 tablespoon freshly minced ginger

- 1/2 teaspoon arrowroot

- 2 boneless chicken breasts, cooked and sliced thinly

Directions:

1. Shred the cabbage with a knife.

2. Slice onion and add to your platter alongside the rotisserie chicken.

3. Add a dollop of mayonnaise on top and drizzle olive oil over the cabbage.

4. Season with sunflower seeds and pepper according to your taste.

5. Enjoy!

Nutrition:

Calories: 368; Fat: 18g; Net Carbohydrates: 8g; Protein: 42g; Fiber: 3g; Carbohydrates: 11g

17.   Hearty Chicken Liver Stew

Preparation: 10 minutes Cooking: 20 minutes Servings: 2

Ingredients:

- 10 ounces chicken livers 1-ounce onion, chopped

- 2 ounces sour cream

- 1 tablespoon olive oil

- Sunflower seeds to taste

Directions:

1. Take a pan and place it over medium heat.

2. Add oil and let it heat up.

3. Add onions and fry until just browned.

4. Add livers and season with sunflower seeds.

5. Cook until livers are half cooked.

6. Transfer the mix to a stew pot.

7. Add sour cream and cook for 20 minutes.

8. Serve and enjoy!

Nutrition:

Calories: 146; Fat: 9g; Carbohydrates: 2g; Protein: 15g

18.   Chicken Quesadilla

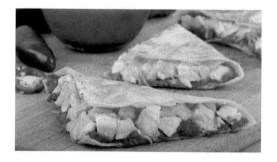

Preparation time: 10 minutes

Cooking time: 35 minutes

Servings: 2

Ingredients:

- ¼ cup ranch dressing

- ½ cup cheddar cheese, shredded

- 20 slices bacon, center-cut

- 2 cups grilled chicken, sliced

Directions:

1. Re-heat your oven to 400 degrees F.

2. Line baking sheet using parchment paper.

3. Weave bacon into two rectangles and bake for 30 minutes.

4. Lay grilled chicken over bacon square, drizzling ranch dressing on top.

5. Sprinkle cheddar cheese and top with another bacon square.

6. Bake for 5 minutes more.

7. Slice and serve.

8. Enjoy!

Nutrition:

Calories: 619, Fat: 35g, Carbohydrates: 2g, Protein: 79g

19. Mustard Chicken

Preparation: 10 minutes Cooking: 40 minutes Servings: 2

Ingredients:

- 2 chicken breasts

- 1/4 cup chicken broth

- 2 tablespoons mustard

- 1 1/2 tablespoons olive oil

- 1/2 teaspoon paprika

- 1/2 teaspoon chili powder

- 1/2 teaspoon garlic powder

Directions:

1. Take a small bowl and mix mustard, olive oil, paprika, chicken broth, garlic powder, chicken broth, and chili.

2. Add chicken breast and marinate for 30 minutes.

3. Take a lined baking sheet and arrange the chicken.

4. Bake for 35 minutes at 375 degrees F.

5. Serve and enjoy!

Nutrition: Calories: 531; Fat: 23g; Carbohydrates: 10g; Protein: 64g

20. Chicken and Carrot Stew

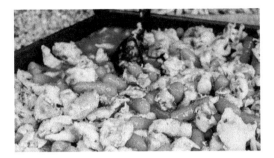

Preparation time: 15 minutes

Cooking time: 6 minutes

Servings: 4

Ingredients:

- 4 boneless chicken breasts, cubed

- 3 cups of carrots, peeled and cubed

- 1 cup onion, chopped

- 1 cup tomatoes, chopped

- 1 teaspoon of dried thyme

- 2 cups of chicken broth

- 2 garlic cloves, minced

- Sunflower seeds and pepper as needed

Directions:

1. Add all of the listed ingredients to a Slow Cooker.

2. Stir and close the lid.

3. Cook for 6 hours.

4. Serve hot and enjoy!

Nutrition: Calories: 182, Fat: 3g, Carbohydrates: 10g, Protein: 39g

21.   The Delish Turkey Wrap

Preparation time: 10 minutes

Cooking time: 10 minutes

Servings: 6

Ingredients:

- 1 ¼ pounds ground turkey, lean

- 4 green onions, minced

- 1 tablespoon olive oil

- 1 garlic clove, minced

- 2 teaspoons chili paste

- 8-ounce water chestnut, diced

- 3 tablespoons hoisin sauce

- 2 tablespoon coconut aminos

- 1 tablespoon rice vinegar

- 12 almond butter lettuce leaves

- 1/8 teaspoon sunflower seeds

Directions:

1. Take a pan and place it over medium heat, add turkey and garlic to the pan.

2. Heat for 6 minutes until cooked.

3. Take a bowl and transfer turkey to the bowl.

4. Add onions and water chestnuts.

5. Stir in hoisin sauce, coconut aminos, and vinegar and chili paste.

6. Toss well and transfer mix to lettuce leaves.

7. Serve and enjoy!

Nutrition:

Calories: 162; Fat: 4g; Net Carbohydrates: 7g; Protein: 23g

22.   Almond butternut Chicken

Preparation time: 15 minutes

Cooking time: 30 minutes

Servings: 4

Ingredients:

- ½ pound Nitrate free bacon

- 6 chicken thighs, boneless and skinless

- 2-3 cups almond butternut squash, cubed

- Extra virgin olive oil

- Fresh chopped sage

- Sunflower seeds and pepper as needed

Directions:

1. Prepare your oven by preheating it to 425 degrees F.

2. Take a large skillet and place it over medium-high heat, add bacon and fry until crispy.

3. Take a slice of bacon and place it on the side, crumble the bacon.

4. Add cubed almond butternut squash in the bacon grease and sauté, season with sunflower seeds and pepper.

5. Once the squash is tender, remove skillet and transfer to a plate.

6. Add coconut oil to the skillet and add chicken thighs, cook for 10 minutes.

7. Season with sunflower seeds and pepper.

8. Remove skillet from stove and transfer to oven.

9. Bake for 12-15 minutes, top with the crumbled bacon and sage.

10. Enjoy!

Nutrition: Calories: 323; Fat: 19g; Carbohydrates: 8g; Protein: 12g

23.   Zucchini Zoodles with Chicken and Basil

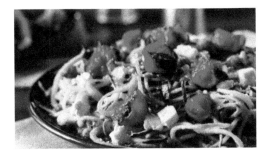

Preparation time: 10 minutes

Cooking time: 10 minutes

Servings: 3

Ingredients:

- 2 chicken fillets, cubed

- 2 tablespoons ghee

- 1-pound tomatoes, diced

- ½ cup basil, chopped

- ¼ cup almond milk

- 1 garlic clove, peeled, minced

- 1 zucchini, shredded

Directions:

1. Sauté cubed chicken in ghee until no longer pink. Add tomatoes and season with sunflower seeds.

2. Simmer and reduce liquid.

3. Prepare your zucchini Zoodles by shredding zucchini in a food processor.

4. Add basil, garlic, coconut almond milk to the chicken and cook for a few minutes. Add half of the zucchini Zoodles to a bowl and top with creamy tomato basil chicken. Enjoy!

Nutrition:

Calories: 540; Fat: 27g; Carbohydrates: 13g; Protein: 59g

24. Duck with Cucumber and Carrots

Preparation time: 10 minutes

Cooking time: 40 minutes

Servings: 8

Ingredients:

- 1 duck, cut up into medium pieces
- 1 chopped cucumber, chopped
- 1 tablespoon low sodium vegetable stock - 2 carrots, chopped
- 2 cups of water
- Black pepper as needed
- 1-inch ginger piece, grated

Directions:

1. Add duck pieces to your Instant Pot.
2. Add cucumber, stock, carrots, water, ginger, pepper and stir.
3. Lock up the lid and cook on LOW pressure for 40 minutes.
4. Release the pressure naturally.
5. Serve and enjoy!

Nutrition: Calories: 206; Fats: 7g; Carbs: 28g; Protein: 16g

25.   Parmesan Baked Chicken

Preparation time: 5 minutes

Cooking time: 20 minutes

Servings: 2

Ingredients:

- 2 tablespoons ghee

- 2 boneless chicken breasts, skinless

- Pink sunflower seeds

- Freshly ground black pepper

- ½ cup mayonnaise, low fat

- ¼ cup parmesan cheese, grated

- 1 tablespoon dried Italian seasoning, low fat, low sodium

- ¼ cup crushed pork rinds

Directions:

1. Preheat your oven to 425 degrees F.

2. Take a large baking dish and coat with ghee.

3. Pat chicken breasts dry and wrap with a towel.

4. Season with sunflower seeds and pepper.

5. Place in baking dish.

6. Take a small bowl and add mayonnaise, parmesan cheese, Italian seasoning.

7. Slather mayo mix evenly over chicken breast.

8. Sprinkle crushed pork rinds on top.

9. Bake for 20 minutes until topping is browned.

10. Serve and enjoy!

Nutrition:

Calories: 850; Fat: 67g; Carbohydrates: 2g; Protein: 60g

CHAPTER 6:

Dinner

26.   Turkey Stir Fry with Vegetables

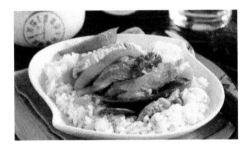

Preparation Time: 10 minutes

Cooking Time: 30 minutes

Servings: 2

Ingredients:

- 1 Cup turkey, cooked, cut into 1/2-inch cubes

- 2 Cups vegetables, fresh or frozen or canned

- 2 cups brown rice, cooked

- 1 Tablespoon oil

- 1/2 teaspoon sugar 1/2 Tablespoon ginger, minced

- 1/4 Teaspoon clove Garlic, minced 1/2 teaspoon salt

Directions:

1. In a non-stick frying pan, heat oil at low-medium temperature.

2. Put the turkey, vegetables, minced ginger, garlic, and salt.

3. Stir and fry for about one minute.

4. Add sugar and continue stirring.

5. Reduce heat to avoid scorching and continue cooking until the vegetables become tender.

6. When the vegetables become tender, remove them from the heat.

7. In the event, if the vegetables did not cook well, pour 2-3 tablespoons of water and cook until it becomes soft.

8. Serve with the cooked rice.

Nutrition:

Calories: 223 Total Fat: 12g Total Carbohydrates: 21g Fiber: 6g

Sugar: 8g Protein: 13g

27. Tuscan White Beans with Shrimp, Spinach, and Feta

Preparation Time: 10 minutes

Cooking Time: 20 minutes

Servings: 2

Ingredients:

1 Pound shrimp, large, peeled, and deveined

15 Ounces cannellini beans, saltless, rinsed and drained

1 1/2 Ounces low-fat feta cheese, shredded

1/2 cup chicken broth, fat-free, low-sodium

4 Cloves clove Garlic, minced

2 Teaspoons sage, fresh, finely chopped

2 Tablespoons balsamic vinegar

2 Tablespoons olive oil

1 medium-size onion, chopped

5 cups baby spinach

Directions:

1. Take a large skillet

2. Pour one tablespoon of olive oil and bring to medium temperature.

3. When the oil becomes hot, put the shrimp for 2-3 minutes.

4. Transfer the shrimp to a plate when its color changes.

5. Pour the balance oil into the skillet and put chopped onion, sage, and garlic.

6. Stir and cook until the onion turns a golden color. Within 4 minutes of cooking, the onion will start to become a golden color.

7. Add vinegar and continue cooking for another half minute.

8. Now add the chicken broth and cook for two minutes until it boils.

9. At this time, add the vegetables and put the spinach. Cook until the spinach starts to wilt.

10. Get the skillet from the heat and put the cooked shrimp and stir.

11. Serve by topping with feta cheese.

Nutrition:

Calories: 280 Total Fat: 7g Total Carbohydrates: 22g

Fiber: 6g Sugar: 0.5g Protein: 32g

28. Chicken & Broccoli in Sesame Noodles

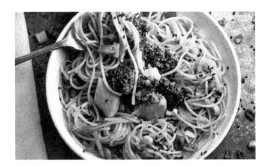

Preparation Time: 5 minutes

Cooking Time: 20 minutes

Servings: 2

Ingredients:

- 1/2 Cup chicken, cooked & diced

- 8 Ounces whole-wheat spaghetti noodles

- 1/4 cup vegetable oil

- 12 Ounces broccoli florets, frozen

- 1 Tablespoon garlic, minced

- 2 Tablespoons sugar

- 2 Tablespoons rice vinegar

- 2 Tablespoons soy sauce, low sodium

- 1 Tablespoon sesame seeds, toasted

Directions:

1. Prepare pasta as per the package instructions and keep it aside.

2. In a medium bowl, whisk soy sauce, sugar, and vinegar and keep aside.

3. Add the oil in a skillet and bring to medium heat.

4. Put broccoli and garlic and cook until it becomes soft.

5. Now add the chicken pieces and cook very well for about 10 minutes.

6. When the chicken's color starts to change, add soy sauce mixture and pasta.

7. Mix it thoroughly.

8. Serve by drizzling sesame seeds on top.

Nutrition:

Calories: 240 Total Fat: 9g

Total Carbohydrates: 27g

Fiber: 4g Sugar: 5g

Protein: 13g

29. Spicy Baked Potatoes

Preparation Time: 10 minutes

Cooking Time: 25 minutes

Servings: 2

Ingredients:

- 4 medium-size sweet potatoes

- 1/3 cups black beans, canned, rinsed and drained

- 1/2 cup Greek yogurt no-fat

- 1 Teaspoon olive oil

- 1 Teaspoon taco seasoning, low sodium

- 1/2 cup red pepper, diced

- 1/2 cup onion, chopped

- 1/2 teaspoon paprika

- 1 teaspoon chili powder   1/2 Teaspoon cumin

- 1/2 cup Mexican cheese, low-fat

- 1/4 teaspoon salt 1/2 cup salsa

Directions:

1. Make holes in the potato with a fork or any sharp kitchen tools.

2. Microwave it for about 8-10 minutes until it becomes tender.

3. In a bowl, mix taco seasoning with yogurt.

4. Now heat oil in a saucepan at medium temperature.

5. Put chopped onions, paprika, chili powder, peppers, cumin, and sauté continuously on medium heat until the onion gets caramelized.

6. Add salt and continue stirring. Wait for about 5 minutes to get the onion caramelized.

7. Now add the drained black beans; continue heating and stirring for about 5 minutes.

8. Using a fork, slice the potato lengthwise.

9. Serve it by dressing with 2 tablespoons of shredded cheese, 2 tablespoons of Greek yogurt mixture, black bean mixture 1/3, and 2 tablespoons of salsa.

Nutrition:

Calories: 260 Total Fat: 15g

Total Carbohydrates: 32g Fiber: 6g

Sugar: 3g Protein: 5g

30. Tandoori Chicken

Preparation Time: 10 minutes

Cooking Time: 20 minutes

Servings: 2

Ingredients:

- 6 Pieces boneless chicken cut into 1-inch pieces

- 1 cup yogurt, plain, fatless

- 2 Tablespoons paprika

- 1 teaspoon yellow curry powder

- 1 teaspoon red pepper, crushed

- 1/2 cup lemon juice

- 5 cloves garlic cloves, minced

- 1 teaspoon ground ginger

- 6 Skewers, soaked in water for 15 minutes

Directions:

1. Using a blender, combine yogurt, garlic, lemon juice, curry powder, red pepper, ginger, and paprika thoroughly until it becomes a smooth paste.

2. Set your over to 390°F and preheat.

3. On the soaked skewers, skew all chicken pieces.

4. Place the skewed chicken on a plain plate and marinate the chicken with the blended mix. Keep the remaining marinade mix for later use.

5. Cover the marinated skewed chicken and refrigerate for a better marinade effect.

6. Let it marinates for about 4 hours and after that, take it out and again brush with the remaining marinade mix.

7. Now, bake it for about 20 minutes or bake it until the chicken's secretion from the chicken stops or the meat gets pierced. Serve hot.

Nutrition:

Calories: 112 Total Fat: 2g

Total Carbohydrates: 11g Fiber: 2g

Sugar: 1g

Protein: 10g

31.   Pork Tenderloin with Sweet Potatoes & Apple

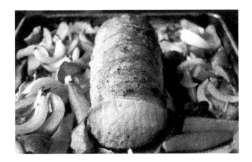

Preparation Time: 10 minutes

Cooking Time: 30 minutes

Servings: 2

Ingredients:

- 12 Ounces of pork tenderloin

- 1 Potato, large, cut into 1/2" cubes

- 3/4 cup apple cider

- 1/4 cup apple cider vinegar

- 1/4 Teaspoon paprika, smoked

- 2 Tablespoons maple syrup

- 1/4 Teaspoon ginger, dried

- 1 Teaspoon ginger, fresh, minced

- 2 Tablespoons vegetable oil

- 1 Apple, cut into 1/2" cube size

Directions:

1. Take a large bowl and start mixing smoked paprika, apple cider, maple syrup, apple cider vinegar, black pepper, ginger, and keep aside.

2. Set your oven to 360°F and preheat.

3. Take a large oven-safe sauté pan and heat oil at medium temperature.

4. Once the oil becomes hot, put the pork tenderloin. Continue cooking at medium temperature for about 10 minutes.

5. Flip sides and make sure to cook all sides evenly. Once the sides cooked well, remove them from the heat.

6. Arrange the sweet potatoes around the tenderloin. Pour apple cider mixture over it.

7. Cover the saucepan and bake it for about 10 minutes.

8. Place the sliced apple pieces around the pork tenderloin and bake for another 10 minutes, until the tenderloin temperature shows 340°F.

9. Once the temperature is reached at 340°F, stop baking and remove the pork tenderloin, potatoes and apple and allow it to settle for 10 minutes.

10. Heat the cider mixture and reduce to 1/4 cup.

11. Slice the pork to edible size. Serve along with sweet potatoes and apples.

12. Dress it with apple cider while serving.

Nutrition:

Calories: 339 Total Fat: 12g

Total Carbohydrates: 21g Fiber: 3g

Sugar: 0g

Protein: 35g

32. Tasty Tortilla Bake

Preparation Time: 15 minutes

Cooking Time: 30 minutes

Servings: 2

Ingredients:

- 8 Tortilla, sliced into half

- 1 cup corn, frozen or fresh

- 1 Onion, green, chopped

- 3 Eggs

- 1 cup milk, fat-free

- 1 cup Monterey Jack cheese

- 1 cup black beans, cooked

- 2 Ounces green chilies, canned, chopped

- 1/2 teaspoon chili powder

- 1 Tomato, sliced

- 1/4 teaspoon salsa

Directions:

1. Take an 8" square shaped baking tray and spray some cooking oil.

2. Set your oven to 370°F and preheat.

3. Layer in 5 tortilla halves in the bottom of the baking pan.

4. Top it with one-third of the cheese, beans, and corn layer by layer. Repeat the layering.

5. Beat egg in a bowl with chili powder, green chili, and milk. Now pour the mix over the tortilla.

6. Dress the tomato slice over the tortilla and spread the remaining cheese on top.

7. Bake it for 30 minutes and check to confirm its baking status.

8. Allow it to settle for another 10 minutes.

9. Serve with salsa.

Nutrition:

Calories: 181

Total Fat: 8g

Total Carbohydrates: 21g

Fiber: 0g

Sugar: 4g

Protein: 4g

CHAPTER 7:

Sides

33.   Tomatoes Side Salad

Preparation: 10 minutes Cooking: 0 minutes Servings: 4

Ingredients:

- ½ bunch mint, chopped

- 8 plum tomatoes, sliced

- 1 teaspoon mustard

- 1 tablespoon rosemary vinegar

- A pinch of black pepper

Directions:

1. In a bowl, mix vinegar with mustard and pepper and whisk.

2. In another bowl, combine the tomatoes with the mint and the vinaigrette, toss, divide between plates and serve as a side dish.

3. Enjoy!

Nutrition: calories 70, fat 2, fiber 2, carbs 6, protein 4

34.   Squash Salsa

Preparation time: 10 minutes

Cooking time: 13 minutes

Servings: 6

Ingredients:

- 3 tablespoons olive oil

- 5 medium squash, peeled and sliced

- 1 cup pepitas, toasted

- 7 tomatillos

- A pinch of black pepper

- 1 small onion, chopped

- 2 tablespoons fresh lime juice

- 2 tablespoons cilantro, chopped

Directions:

1. Heat up a pan over medium heat, add tomatillos, onion and black pepper, stir, cook for 3 minutes, transfer to your food processor and pulse.

2. Add lime juice and cilantro, pulse again and transfer to a bowl.

3. Heat up your kitchen grill over high heat, drizzle the oil over squash slices, grill them for 10 minutes, divide them between plates, add pepitas and tomatillos mix on top and serve as a side dish. Enjoy!

Nutrition: calories 120, fat 2, fiber 1, carbs 7, protein 1

35. Apples and Fennel Mix

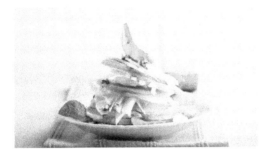

Preparation time: 10 minutes

Cooking time: 0 minutes

Servings: 3

Ingredients:

- 3 big apples, cored and sliced

- 1 and ½ cup fennel, shredded

- 1/3 cup coconut cream

- 3 tablespoons apple vinegar

- ½ teaspoon caraway seeds

- Black pepper to the taste

Directions:

1. In a bowl, mix fennel with apples and toss.

2. In another bowl, mix coconut cream with vinegar, black pepper and caraway seeds, whisk well, add over the fennel mix, toss, divide between plates and serve as a side dish.

3. Enjoy!

Nutrition: calories 130, fat 3, fiber 6, carbs 10, protein 3

36.　Simple Roasted Celery Mix

Preparation time: 10 minutes

Cooking time: 25 minutes

Servings: 3

Ingredients:

- 3 celery roots, cubed

- 2 tablespoons olive oil

- A pinch of black pepper

- 2 cups natural and unsweetened apple juice

- ¼ cup parsley, chopped

- ¼ cup walnuts, chopped

Directions:

1. In a baking dish, combine the celery with the oil, pepper, parsley, walnuts and apple juice, toss to coat, introduce in the oven at 450 degrees F, bake for 25 minutes, divide between plates and serve as a side dish.

2. Enjoy!

Nutrition: calories 140, fat 2, fiber 2, carbs 7, protein 7

37.   Thyme Spring Onions Cooking time: 40 minutes

Servings: 8

Ingredients:

- 15 spring onions

- A pinch of black pepper

- 1 teaspoon thyme, chopped

- 1 tablespoon olive oil

Directions:

1. Put onions in a baking dish, add thyme, black pepper and oil, toss, bake in the oven at 350 degrees F for 40 minutes, divide between plates and serve as a side dish.

2. Enjoy!

Nutrition: calories 120, fat 2, fiber 2, carbs 7, protein 2

38.   Carrot Slaw

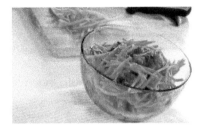

Preparation time: 10 minutes Cooking time: 10 minutes

Servings: 4

Ingredients:

- ¼ yellow onion, chopped

- 5 carrots, cut into thin matchsticks

- 1 tablespoon olive oil

- 1 garlic clove, minced

- 1 tablespoon Dijon mustard

- 1 tablespoon red vinegar

- A pinch of black pepper

- 1 tablespoon lemon juice

Directions:

1. In a bowl, mix vinegar with black pepper, mustard and lemon juice and whisk.

2. Heat up a pan with the oil over medium heat, add onion, stir and cook for 5 minutes.

3. Add garlic and carrots, stir, cook for 5 minutes more, transfer to a salad bowl, cool down, add the vinaigrette, toss, divide between plates and serve as a side dish.

4. Enjoy!

Nutrition: calories 120, fat 3, fiber 3, carbs 7, protein 5

39. Watermelon Tomato Salsa

Preparation time: 10 minutes Cooking time: 0 minutes

Servings: 16

Ingredients:

- 4 yellow tomatoes, seedless and chopped

- A pinch of black pepper

- 1 cup watermelon, seedless and chopped

- 1/3 cup red onion, chopped

- 2 jalapeno peppers, chopped

- ¼ cup cilantro, chopped

- 3 tablespoons lime juice

Directions:

1. In a bowl, mix tomatoes with watermelon, onion and jalapeno.

2. Add cilantro, lime juice and pepper, toss, divide between plates and serve as a side dish.

3. Enjoy!

Nutrition: calories 87, fat 1, fiber 2, carbs 4, protein 7

40.   Edamame Side Salad

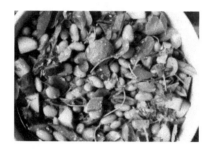

Preparation time: 10 minutes Cooking time: 0 minutes

Servings: 4

Ingredients:

- 1 tablespoon ginger, grated

- 2 green onions, chopped

- 3 cups edamame, blanched

- 2 tablespoons rice vinegar

- 1 tablespoon sesame seeds

Directions:

1. In a bowl, combine the ginger with the onions, edamame, vinegar and sesame seeds, toss, divide between plates and serve as a side dish. Enjoy!

Nutrition: calories 120, fat 3, fiber 2, carbs 5, protein 9

41.   Tomato and Avocado Salad

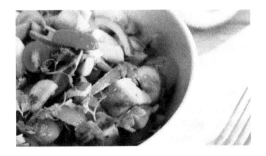

Preparation time: 10 minutes Cooking time: 0 minutes

Servings: 4

Ingredients:

- 1 cucumber, chopped

- 1-pound tomatoes, chopped

- 2 avocados, pitted, peeled and chopped

- 1 small red onion, sliced

- 2 tablespoons olive oil

- 2 tablespoons lemon juice

- ¼ cup cilantro, chopped

- Black pepper to the taste

Directions:

1. In a salad bowl, mix tomatoes with onion, avocado, cucumber and cilantro.

2. In a small bowl, mix oil with lemon juice and black pepper, whisk well, pour this over the salad, toss and serve as a side dish.

3. Enjoy!

Nutrition: calories 120, fat 2, fiber 2, carbs 3, protein 4

CHAPTER 8:

Vegetables

42.   Cauliflower Pizza Crust

Preparation time: 15 minutes

Cooking time: 20 minutes

Servings: 6

Ingredients:

- 2 cups cauliflower, chopped

- 1 egg, whisked

- 1 teaspoon butter

- 1 teaspoon dried basil

- 1 teaspoon salt

- 6 oz Cheddar cheese, shredded

- 1 tablespoon heavy cream

Directions:

1. Place the cauliflower in the food processor and blend until you get cauliflower rice.

2. Then squeeze the juice from the cauliflower rice.

3. Line the baking tray with the parchment and then spread parchment with the butter.

4. Place the cauliflower rice in the tray in the shape of the pizza crust.

5. BAKE THE CAULIFLOWER PIZZA CRUST FOR 10 MINUTES AT 365F.

6. Meanwhile, mix up together salt, shredded Cheddar cheese, heavy cream, and egg.

7. When the cauliflower crust is cooked, spread it with cheese mixture and flatten gently it.

8. Bake the meal for 10 minutes more at 375F.

9. When the pizza crust is cooked, cut it into 6 servings.

Nutrition: calories 147, fat 11.7, fiber 0.8, carbs 2.3, protein 8.7

43. Zucchini Ravioli

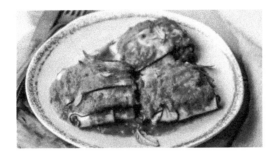

Preparation time: 20 minutes

Cooking time: 15 minutes

Servings: 4

Ingredients:

- 1 zucchini, trimmed

- 2 tablespoons ricotta cheese

- ½ cup spinach, chopped

- 1 teaspoon olive oil

- ½ teaspoon salt

- 1/3 cup marinara sauce

- 4 oz Parmesan, grated

Directions:

1. Slice the zucchini with the help of the peeler to get long slices.

2. Then take 4 zucchini slices and make the cross from them.

3. Repeat the same steps with all remaining zucchini slices.

4. After this, place chopped spinach in the skillet. Add salt and olive oil. Mix up spinach and cook it for 5 minutes. Stir it from time to time. After this, mix up spinach with ricotta and stir well.

5. Pour marinara sauce in the casserole dish.

6. Place the ricotta mixture in the center of every zucchini cross and fold up them.

7. Transfer zucchini balls -ravioli in the casserole to dish on the marinara sauce. Sprinkle the zucchini ravioli over with grated Parmesan and transfer the casserole dish in the preheated to the 395F oven. Cook the meal for 15 minutes.

Nutrition: calories 141, fat 8.9, fiber 1.2, carbs 5.9, protein 11.1

44.   Crunchy Okra Bites

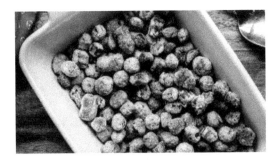

Preparation time: 10 minutes

Cooking time: 12 minutes

Servings: 2

Ingredients:

- 1 cup okra, roughly sliced

- ¼ cup almond flour

- 1 tablespoon coconut flakes

- 1 teaspoon chili powder

- ½ teaspoon salt

- 3 eggs, whisked

Directions:

1. In the mixing bowl, mix up together almond flour, coconut flakes, chili powder, and salt.

2. Place the sliced okra into the whisked egg and mix up well.

3. Then coat every okra bite into the almond flour mixture.

4. Line the tray with the parchment.

5. Place the okra bites into the tray to make the okra layer.

6. Preheat the oven to 375F.

7. Place the tray with okra bites in the oven and cook for 12 minutes. Chill the hot okra bites little before serving.

Nutrition: calories 147, fat 9.5, fiber 2.7, carbs 6.1, protein 10.3

45.   Vegan Moussaka

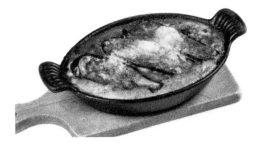

Preparation time: 15 minutes

Cooking time: 35 minutes

Servings: 88

Ingredients:

- 2 eggplants, trimmed

- 1 white onion, chopped

- 1 garlic clove, diced

- ¼ cup tomatoes, crushed

- ½ teaspoon ground cinnamon

- 1 teaspoon salt

- 1 teaspoon ground black pepper

- 1 teaspoon ground paprika

- 2 tablespoons coconut oil

- 2 tablespoons ricotta cheese

- 1 oz Cheddar cheese, shredded

- 1 tablespoon heavy cream

Directions:

1. Place the coconut oil in the saucepan and melt it.

2. Meanwhile, chop the eggplants.

3. Place the eggplants and onion in the hot coconut oil. Add diced garlic.

4. Mix up the vegetables and cook them for 10 minutes or until they start to be soft.

5. MEANWHILE, MIX UP TOGETHER HEAVY CREAM, RICOTTA CHEESE, AND SHREDDED CHEDDAR CHEESE.

6. Transfer the roasted vegetables in the blender and blend for 3 minutes or until they are smooth.

7. After this, add all spices and crushed tomatoes, Blend the mixture 1 minute more.

8. Transfer the eggplant mixture in the casserole dish and flatten it well with the help of the spatula.

9. Place ricotta mixture over the eggplant mixture.

10. Bake moussaka for 20 minutes at the preheated to the 360F oven.

11. Chill the cooked meal for 10 minutes before serving.

Nutrition: calories 99, fat 5.9, fiber 5.5, carbs 10.4, protein 3

21 Days Meal Plan

DAY	BREAKFAST	LUNCH	DINNER
1	Shrimp Skillet	Curried Chicken wrap	Shrimp Cocktail
2	Coconut Yogurt with Chia Seeds	Open-Faced Garden Tuna Sandwich	Quinoa and Scallops Salad
3	Chia Pudding	Baked Macaroni	Squid and Shrimp Salad
4	Egg Fat Bombs	Zucchini Pad Thai	Parsley Seafood Cocktail
5	Morning "Grits	Easy Roasted Salmon	Shrimp and Onion Ginger Dressing
6	Scotch Eggs	Shrimp with Pasta, Artichoke, and Spinach	Fruit Shrimp Soup
7	Bacon Sandwich	Pistachio Crusted Halibut with Spicy Yogurt	Mussels and Chickpea Soup
8	Noatmeal	Paella with Chicken, Leeks, and Tarragon	Fish Stew
9	Breakfast Bake with Meat	Roasted Brussels Sprouts, Chicken, and Potatoes	Shrimp and Broccoli Soup
10	Breakfast	Shepherd's Pie	Coconut Turkey Mix
11	Egg and Vegetable Hash	Salmon and Edamame Cakes	Lime Shrimp and Kale
12	Cowboy Skillet	Flat Bread Pizza	Parsley Cod Mix
13	Feta Quiche	Spinach Salad with Walnuts and Strawberry	Salmon and Cabbage Mix

14	Bacon Pancakes	Chicken Vegetable Soup	Decent Beef and Onion Stew
15	Waffles	Avocado Sandwich with Lemon and Cilantro	Clean Parsley and Chicken Breast
16	Rolled Omelette with Mushrooms	Tofu and Mushroom Burger	Zucchini Beef Sauté with Coriander Greens
17	Quiche Lorraine	Cobb Salad	Hearty Lemon and Pepper Chicken
18	Breakfast Zucchini Bread	Veggie Sushi	Walnuts and Asparagus Delight
19	Granola	Curried Chicken wrap	Healthy Carrot Chips
20	Cheddar Souffle	Open-Faced Garden Tuna Sandwich	Beef Soup
21	Mediterranean Omelette	Baked Macaroni	Shrimp Cocktail

Conclusion

The Dash Diet is designed to help ladies lose weight and stay healthy. There are many useful tips and easy recipes in this cookbook that can help you better understand the Dash Diet and make healthy food choices.

Even if you aren't following the Dash Diet, this cookbook can help you need a well-made, delicious meal. At Dash Diet, we understand that our products' quality is just as important as the quality of our products. That is why Dash Diet uses hardened steel components for its ratchets.

Our ratchets are made with hardened steel that is hand-polished and handcrafted by experts in the USA. This ensures a long life for your new tool. Each part is made with precision to ensure a strong bond between the ratchet tool's male and female heads. Most people don't use their kitchen knives for cooking. Most people don't know that you should always wash them after cutting something, primarily if you've used a grinder on them.